Dyslexia

Bringing out the Best in Dyslexic Kids and Unlocking the

Hidden Potential of the Dyslexic Brain

Bill Sam

ISBN: 978-1-63750-202-0

Table of Contents

Introduction

"A must read for parents, educators, and people with dyslexia."

Did you know that many successful architects, lawyers, engineers—even bestselling novelists—had difficulties learning to read and write as children? In this groundbreaking book, Bill Sam explain how 20% of people—individuals with dyslexia—share a unique learning style that can create advantages in a classroom, at a job, or at home.

Understanding brain imaging, the symptoms, strength of people with dyslexia among many other factors are important solution to understanding and bringing out the best in dyslexic people.

For kids with an official dyslexia diagnosis, or kids

struggling with dyslexia related symptoms, learning to read can be challenging. Using a targeted approach to skill development, Learning to Read for Kids with Dyslexia applies the latest research-based learning methods to games and activities that strengthen auditory discrimination skills, support letter formation in writing, and most importantly—make reading fun.

Using their combined expertise in neurology and education, the authors show how these individuals not only perceive the written word differently but may also excel at spatial reasoning, see insightful connections that others simply miss, understand the world in stories, and display amazing creativity. Blending personal stories with hard science, This book has an invaluable advice on how parents, educators, and individuals with dyslexia can recognize and use the strengths of the dyslexic learning style in: material reasoning (used by architects and engineers); interconnected reasoning (scientists and designers), narrative reasoning (novelists and lawyers); and dynamic reasoning (economists and entrepreneurs.)

With prescriptive advice and inspiring testimonials, this paradigm-shifting book proves that dyslexia doesn't have to be a detriment, but can often become an asset for success.

Chapter 1

What to Know About Dyslexia

Dyslexia can be an often-misunderstood, confusing term for reading problems. The term dyslexia comprises of two different parts: **dys-** *abnormal, or impaired* or *difficult*, and **-lexia** signifying *words, reading, or vocabulary*. So quite actually, *dyslexia* means difficulty with words (Catts & Kamhi, 2005).

Regardless of the many confusions and misunderstandings, the word dyslexia is often utilized by medical personnel, researchers, and clinicians. Among the most typical misunderstandings concerning this condition is that dyslexia is an issue of attention, or term reversals (b/d, was/noticed) or of characters, words, or sentences "dance around" on the web page (Rayner,

Foorman, Perfetti, Pesetsky, & Seidenberg, 2001).

Actually, writing and reading words backwards are normal in the first stages of understanding how to read and write among average and dyslexic children as well, and the existence of reversals may or might not indicate an underlying reading problem.

Probably one of the most complete definitions of dyslexia originates from over twenty years of research:

- Dyslexia is a particular learning impairment that is neurobiological in the source. It is seen as a problem with accurate and/or fluent phrase acknowledgement, and poor spelling and decoding capabilities. These troubles typically derive from a deficit in the phonological element of vocabulary that is often unpredicted with regards to other cognitive skills and the provision of effective classroom training. (Lyon, Shaywitz, & Shaywitz, 2003)

- Dyslexia is a particular learning impairment in reading that often impacts spelling as well. Actually, reading impairment is the most common and most carefully analysed study of the training disabilities, influencing 80% (eighty percent) of most specified learning disabilities. As a result of this, we use the conditions: *dyslexia and reading disabilities* (RD) interchangeably in this specific article to spell it out to the students.

It really is neurobiological in origins, and therefore the problem is situated physically in the mind. Dyslexia is not triggered by poverty, developmental hold off, conversation, hearing impairments, or learning another vocabulary, although those conditions may put a kid more in danger of creating a reading impairment (Snow, Burns, & Griffin, 1998).

Children with dyslexia will most likely show two apparent problems when asked to learn text message at their quality level. First, they'll not have the ability to read much of the text message; you will see many words which they'll stumble, think of, or try to "audio out." This is actually the problem with *"fluent term recognition"* identified in the last definition.

Second, they will show decoding difficulties, and therefore their attempts to recognize words they don't know will produce many mistakes. They'll not be very accurate in using letter-sound associations in mixture with context to recognize unknown words.

These problems in phrase recognition are credited to a

fundamental deficit in the sound element of language, that means it is very hard for readers connecting characters and sounds to be able to decode. People who have dyslexia frequently have trouble comprehending what they read because of the fantastic difficulty they experience in accessing the imprinted words.

Common Misunderstandings about Students with Reading Disabilities

- Writing words backwards are symptoms of dyslexia.

- Writing characters and words backwards are normal in the first stages of understanding how to read and write among average and dyslexic children. It is an indicator that orthographic representations (i.e. forms and spellings of words) have never been firmly founded, and a child with this characteristic commonly has reading impairment (Adams, 1990).

Reading disabilities are triggered by visual belief problems.

The existing consensus predicated on a big body of research (e.g., Lyon et al., 2003; Morris et al., 1998; Rayner et al., 2001; Wagner & Torgesen, 1987) is that dyslexia is most beneficially characterized as a problem with vocabulary digesting at the phoneme level, with no problem with visual digesting.

In the event that you just provide them with plenty of time, children will outgrow dyslexia.

There is absolutely no evidence that dyslexia is a problem that may be outgrown. There is certainly, however, strong proof that children with reading problems show an ongoing prolonged deficit in their reading, rather than simply developing later like average children (Francis, Shaywitz, Stuebing, Shaywitz, & Fletcher, 1996). More strong proof demonstrates that children with dyslexia continue steadily to experience reading problems into adolescence and adulthood (Shaywitz et al., 1999, 2003).

More males than ladies have dyslexia.

Longitudinal research implies that as much girls as boys are influenced by dyslexia (Shaywitz, Shaywitz, Fletcher, & Escobar, 1990). There are numerous possible known reasons for the over identification of men by colleges, including higher behavioural performance and a smaller capability to play among kids. More research is required to determine why.

Dyslexia only impacts people who speak British.

Dyslexia appears in every cultures and dialects in the world with written vocabulary, including the ones that do not use an alphabetic script such as Korean and Hebrew. In British, the principal difficulty is accurate decoding of unfamiliar words. In constant orthographies such as German or Italian, dyslexia shows up more regularly as a problem with fluent reading - people may be accurate, but very decrease (Ziegler & Goswami, 2005).

People who have dyslexia will reap the benefits of coloured text message overlays or lens.

There is absolutely no strong research evidence that mentioned using coloured overlays or special lens has any influence on the term reading or comprehension of children with dyslexia (American Optometric Association, 2004; Iovino, Fletcher, Breitmeyer, &

Foorman, 1998).

A person with dyslexia can't ever figure out how to read.

This is not true. The sooner children who struggle are recognized and provided organized, intense teaching, the less severe their problems will tend to be (Country wide Institute of Child Health insurance and Human Being Development, 2000; Torgesen, 2002). With properly intensive instructions, however, even teenagers with dyslexia may become accurate, albeit decrease people (Torgesen et al., 2001).

What regions of the mind relate with language and reading?

The mind is a complex organ that has many different functions. It sets the body and receives, analyses, and stores information.

The brain can be divided down the centre lengthwise into the right and a left hemisphere. A lot of the areas accountable for talk, language digesting, and reading are in the left hemisphere, and because of this we will concentrate our explanations and numbers on the still left side of the brain. Within each hemisphere, we find the next four brain lobes.

The frontal lobe is the biggest and accountable for controlling speech, reasoning, planning, regulating emotions, and consciousness.

In the 19th century, Paul Broca was discovering areas of the mind used for language and observed a particular area of the brain that was impaired in a guy whose speech became limited after a stroke. This area received increasingly more attention, now we realize that Broca's area, located within the frontal lobe, is very important to the organization, creation, and manipulation of vocabulary and conversation (Joseph, Noble, & Eden, 2001). Regions of the frontal lobe are also very important to silent reading skills (Shaywitz et al., 2002).

The parietal lobe is situated farther behind the brain and controls sensory perceptions as well as linking spoken and written language to memory to provide it meaning so we can know very well what we hear and read.

The occipital lobe, at the trunk of the head, is where in fact the primary visual cortex is situated. Among other styles of visual understanding, the visible cortex is important in the recognition of letters.

The temporal lobe is situated in the lower area of the brain, parallel with the ears, and it is involved with verbal memory.

Wernicke's area, long regarded as important in understanding vocabulary (Joseph et al., 2001), is situated here. This region, determined by Carl Wernicke at a comparable time and using the same methods as Broca, is crucial in language digesting and reading.

Furthermore, converging evidence shows that two other systems, which process vocabulary within and between lobes, are essential for reading.

The foremost is the left *parieto-temporal* system that are involved with word analysis - the conscious, effortful decoding of words (Shaywitz et al., 2002). This region is crucial along the way of mapping words and written words onto their audio correspondences - notice noises and spoken words (Heim & Keil, 2004). This area is also very important to comprehending written and spoken vocabulary (Joseph et al., 2001).

The next system that is very important to reading is the still left *occipito-temporal* area. This technique appears to be involved in automated, rapid usage of whole words and it is a crucial area for skilled, fluent reading (Shaywitz et al., 2002, 2004).

Exactly what does brain imaging research reveal about dyslexia?

Structural brain differences

Studies of structural variations in the brains of individuals of all age groups show distinctions between people who have and without reading disabilities.

The brain is chiefly composed of two types: *grey matter and white matter*. *Grey matter* is exactly what we see whenever we take a look at a brain and is mainly made up of nerve cells. Its main function is digesting information.

White matter is available within the deeper elements of the mind, and comprises of connective fibres protected in myelin, the coating made to facilitate communication between nerves. *White matter* is mainly accountable for information transfer in the brain.

Booth and Burman (2001) found that individuals with dyslexia have less grey matter in the left parieto-temporal area than non-dyslexic individuals. Having less grey matter in this area of the brain may lead to problems digesting the sound framework of vocabulary (phonological consciousness).

Many people who have dyslexia likewise have less white matter in this same area than average readers, which is important because more white matter is correlated with an increase of reading skill (Deutsch, Dougherty, Bammer, Siok, Gabrieli, & Wandell, 2005). Having less white matter could lessen the power or efficiency of the parts of the brain to talk to one another.

Other structural analyses of the brains of individuals with and without RD have found variations in hemispherical asymmetry. Specifically, most brains of right-handed, non-dyslexic people are asymmetrical with the still left hemisphere being bigger than the same area on the right.

On the other hand, Heim and Keil (2004) discovered that right-handed people who have dyslexia show a pattern of symmetry (right equals left) or asymmetry in the other direction (right bigger than left). The precise reason behind these size variations is the main topic of ongoing research, however they appear to be implicated in the reading and spelling problems of individuals with dyslexia.

Chapter 2

What Can Cause Dyslexia?

Dyslexia is not really a disease; it's a disorder from birth, and it often happens in families. People who have dyslexia aren't stupid or sluggish. Most have average or above-average cleverness, plus they work very hard to conquer their learning problems.

Research shows that dyslexia is really because of the sort of brain information. Pictures of the brain show that whenever people who have dyslexia read, they use various areas of the brain than people without dyslexia. These pictures also show that the brains of individuals with dyslexia don't work effectively during reading. So that is why reading seems like such sluggish, hard work.

What goes on in Dyslexia?

Most people believe that dyslexia causes people to change letters and figures and read words backwards. But reversals happen as a standard part of development, and have emerged in many kids until first or second stage.

The primary problem in dyslexia is trouble recognizing phonemes. They are the basic sound of conversation (the "b" audio in "bat" is a phoneme), so it is a struggle to help make the connection between your audio and notice symbol for the sound, and also to blend sound into words.

This makes it hard to identify short, familiar words or even to sound out longer words. It requires lots of time for a person with dyslexia to audio out a term because term reading takes additional time and concentration. A person with dyslexia is often lost during term reading, and reading understanding is poor.

It isn't surprising that individuals with dyslexia have trouble spelling. In addition, they may have trouble expressing themselves on paper and even speaking. Dyslexia is a vocabulary processing disorder, so it makes a difference in all types of vocabulary: spoken or written.

Some individuals have milder kinds of dyslexia, so they could have less trouble in the areas of spoken and written vocabulary. Some individuals work around their dyslexia, but it requires a great deal of effort and further work. Dyslexia isn't something that goes away completely or a person just outgrows. Luckily, with proper help, most people who have dyslexia figure out how to read. They often times find various ways to learn and use those strategies almost all their lives.

Can Dyslexia be cured?

In short, **No.** Dyslexia is a lifelong condition that impacts people into later years. However, that does not mean that education cannot remediate a few of the affected people who have dyslexia with written vocabulary. A big body of proof shows what forms of training struggling readers have to be successful (e.g., Country wide Institute of Child Health insurance and Individual Development, 2000; Snow et al., 1998; Torgesen, 2000).

Now analysts can also "look" inside the brains of children before and after a rigorous intervention and find out for the very first time the consequences of the intervention on the brain activity of children with RD.

Listed below are two such studies.

Aylward et al. (2003) imaged ten children with dyslexia and eleven average people before and after a twenty-eight-hour treatment that only the students with dyslexia received. They likened the two sets of students on out-of-magnet reading assessments as well as the amount of activation during duties of identifying notice sounds.

They discovered that as the control children showed no distinctions between two imaging, the students who received the procedure showed a substantial upsurge in activation, in the areas very important to reading and language through the phonological task. Prior to the intervention, the kids with RD demonstrated significant under-activation in these areas when compared with the control children, and following the treatment, their profiles were virtually identical.

These results must be looked at with caution because of

several limitations. One restriction is having less specificity about the involvement that was provided, another is the tiny test size, and the last is having less an experimental control group (i.e., several children with RD who didn't have the treatment). Lacking any experimental control group, we cannot ensure that the treatment triggered the changes within the brain activation because of so a great many other possible explanations.

Shaywitz et al. (2004) resolved these restrictions in their analysis of brain activation changes before and after an involvement. They examined seventy-eight second and third graders with reading disabilities who had been randomly designated to three organizations:

- the experimental intervention.

- school-based remedial programs.

- Control.

What it's like to have Dyslexia?

When you have dyslexia, it's likely you have trouble reading even simple words you've seen often. You almost certainly will read gradually and believe that you have to work extra hard when reading. You may mix in the letters in short - for example, reading the term "now" as "received" or "left" as "experienced". Words could also blend collectively and areas are lost.

It's likely you have trouble remembering what you've read. You might remember easier when the same information is read for you or you hear it. Phrase problems in mathematics may be especially hard, even if you have mastered the fundamentals of arithmetic.

If you are doing a demonstration before the class, it's likely you have trouble discovering the right words or names for various objects. Spelling and writing usually are extremely hard for individuals with dyslexia.

How is Dyslexia Diagnosed

People who have dyslexia often find ways to work around with their impairment, so nobody will know they're having difficulty. This might save some embarrassment, but getting help will make school and reading easier. Many people are diagnosed as kids, but it isn't unusual for teens or even adults to be diagnosed.

A teen's parents or educators might suspect dyslexia if indeed they notice several problems:

- poor reading skills, despite having normal intelligence.

- poor spelling and writing skills.

- trouble finishing projects and checks within time limits.

- difficulty keeping in mind the right brands for things.

- trouble memorizing written lists and telephone numbers.

- issues with directions (informing right from still left or up from down) or reading maps.

- trouble getting through Spanish classes

Having one of the problems doesn't imply one has dyslexia. But a person who shows many of these indications should be examined for the problem.

A physical exam, including hearing and eyesight tests,

will be achieved to eliminate any medical problems. A college psychologist or learning specialist should give several standardized tests to measure language, reading, spelling, and writing abilities. Sometimes a test of thinking ability (IQ test) is given. Some individuals with dyslexia have trouble in other school skills, like handwriting and math, or they could have trouble attending to or remembering things; if this is actually the case, other types of testing might be achieved.

How to Cope with Dyslexia

Although dealing with dyslexia can be difficult, help is available. Under federal government law, someone identified as having a learning impairment like dyslexia is eligible for extra help from the general public school system. A kid or teen with dyslexia usually must utilize a specially trained teacher, tutor, or reading specialist to understand how to learn and spell better.

The best kind of help teaches knowing of speech sounds in words (called phonemic awareness) and letter-sound correspondences (called phonics). The instructor or teacher should use special learning and practice activities for dyslexia.

Students with dyslexia gets additional time to complete assignments or tests, permission to record class lectures, or copies of lecture notes. Utilizing a computer with spelling checkers are a good idea for written assignments. For older students in challenging classes, services can be by offering recorded versions of any book, even textbooks. Software applications that "reads" printed material aloud is also available, ask your parent, teacher, or learning disability services coordinator ways to get these services if you want them.

Emotional support is vital. People who have dyslexia often get frustrated because no matter how hard they try; they cannot seem to maintain with other students. They could believe that they're much less smart as their peers, and could hide their problems by performing up in course or being the course clown. They could make an effort to get other students to do their work to them. They could pretend that they don't really value their grades or that they think school is dumb.

Relatives and buddies can help people who have dyslexia by knowing that they aren't stupid or lazy, and they should try as hard as they can. It is critical to identify and appreciate each person's talents, whether they're in sports activities, drama, art, creative problem solving, or another thing.

People who have dyslexia shouldn't feel small in their academics or career choices. Most colleges make special accommodations for students with dyslexia, offering them trained tutors, learning aids, software applications, recorded reading assignments, and special arrangements for exams. People who have dyslexia may become doctors, politicians, corporate executives, actors, musicians, artists, teachers, inventors, entrepreneurs, or other things that they choose. Many celebrities with dyslexia have very successful careers in these and other fields, despite having had reading struggles in school.

Chapter 3

Symptoms of Dyslexia

Indicators of dyslexia can be difficult to identify before your son or daughter enters school, however, many early clues may indicate a problem. Once your son or daughter reaches school age, your son or daughter's teacher may be the first to ever notice a problem. Severity varies, however, the condition often becomes apparent as a kid starts understanding how to read.

Before School

Signs a youngster may be vulnerable to dyslexia include:

- Late talking

- Learning new words slowly.

- Problems forming words correctly, such as reversing sound in words or confusing words that sound alike.

- Problems keeping in mind or naming words, digits and colours.

- Difficulty learning nursery rhymes or taking part in rhyming games.

School Age

Once your son or daughter is in college, dyslexia signs or symptoms could become more apparent, including:

- Reading well below the expected level for age.

- Problems controling and understanding what she

or he hears.

- Difficulty discovering the right phrase or forming answers to questions.

- Problems keeping in mind the series of things.

- Difficulty viewing (and occasionally hearing) similarities and variations in characters and words.

- Inability to voice out the pronunciation of a new word.

- Difficulty spelling.

- Spending an unusually very long time completing tasks that involve reading or writing.

- Staying away from activities that involve reading

Teenagers and Adults.

Dyslexia symptoms in teenagers and adults act like those in children. Some typically common dyslexia signs or symptoms in teenagers and adults include:

- Difficulty reading, including reading aloud.

- Sluggish and labour-intensive reading and writing

- Problems spelling.

- Staying away from activities that involve reading

- Mispronouncing titles or words, or problems retrieving words.

- Trouble understanding jokes or expressions which have a meaning not easily comprehended from the precise words (idioms).

- Spending an unusually very long time completing tasks that involve reading or writing.

- Difficulty summarizing a tale.

- Trouble learning a Spanish.

- Difficulty memorizing.

- Difficulty doing mathematics problems

When to see a Medical Expert

Though most children will be ready to learn reading at kindergarten or first grade, children with dyslexia often can't grasp the fundamentals of reading by that point. Talk with your physician if your son or daughter's reading level is below what's expected with regards to age group, or if you see other signals of dyslexia.

When dyslexia goes undiagnosed and untreated, child's years of reading difficulties continue into adulthood.

Request a scheduled appointment at Mayo Clinic

Risk Factors of Dyslexia

Dyslexia risk factors include:

- A family background of dyslexia or other learning disabilities.

- Premature delivery or low delivery weight.

- Exposure during being pregnant to smoking, drugs, alcoholic beverages or contamination that may alter brain development in the foetus.

- Individual distinctions in the elements of the brain that allow reading

- Complications.

Dyslexia can result in lots of problems, including:

- **Trouble learning:** Because reading is an art basic

to many other school topics, a kid with dyslexia reaches a disadvantage generally in most classes and could have trouble maintaining peers.

- **<u>Social problems:</u>** Left untreated, dyslexia can lead to low self-esteem, behavioural problems, stress, aggression, and drawback from friends, parents and instructors.

- **<u>Problems as adults</u>**: The shortcoming to learn and comprehend can prevent a kid from reaching his/her potential as the kid grows up. This may have long-term educational, interpersonal and economic outcomes.

- Children who have dyslexia are in increased threat of having *attention-deficit/hyperactivity disorder (ADHD)*, and vice versa. **ADHD** can cause difficulty sustaining attention as well as hyperactivity and impulsive behaviour, which will make dyslexia harder to take care of.

Common Dyslexia Symptoms

Children can start to show indicators of a learning impairment as soon as preschool years. Whilst every case of dyslexia is exclusive to the average person, there are numerous common characteristics and behaviours of the dyslexic. We've compiled a summary of twenty of the most typical dyslexia symptoms to help you identify if your son or daughter reaches risk level.

Take into account that several are symptoms of dyslexia, not factors behind dyslexia. They are outlined in no particular order.

- Problems with reading.

- Difficulty spelling words on paper products.

- Low Self-confidence or behavioural problems.

- Letter and/or quantity reversals (transposing).

- Issues with pronunciation.

- Omitting sound or words when reading and writing.

- Issues of headaches.

- Difficulty reading aloud.

- Confusion left and right.

- Issues with writing tools like pencils or pens.

- Trouble with sequenced instructions.

- Guessing, skipping or updating words rather than sounding out.

- Strong dental comprehension and poor reading comprehension.

- Letters on a full page may actually move, appear "blurry" or "out of place".

- Difficulty with business and time management.

- Failure to differentiate talk sounds.

- Difficulty repeating phrases or sentences.

- Humiliated by grades.

- Flash credit cards and memorization don't work.

- Reading below quality level or peers

Chapter 4

Brain Imaging

Several techniques can be found to visualize brain anatomy and function. A widely used tool is **magnetic resonance imaging (MRI),** which creates images that can reveal information about brain anatomy (e.g., *the quantity of grey and white matter, the integrity of white matter), brain metabolites (chemicals found in the brain for communication between brain cells), and brain function (where large pools of neurons are energetic*). Functional MRI (fMRI) is dependent on the physiological theory that works in the brain (where neurons are "firing") is associated with a rise of blood circulation compared to that specific area of the brain. The MRI sign bears indirect information about raises in blood circulation. From this transmission, researchers infer the positioning and amount of activity that is associated with an activity, such as reading solitary words, that the study participants are carrying out in the scanner. Data from these studies are usually collected on groupings of individuals rather than individuals for research purposes, only-not to diagnose people with dyslexia.

Which Brain areas get excited about Reading?

Since reading is a cultural invention that arose following the evolution of modern humans, no location within the brain acts as a reading center. Instead, brain locations that sub serve other functions, such as spoken vocabulary and object identification, are redirected (rather than innately given) for the intended purpose of reading (Dehaene & Cohen, 2007). Reading entails multiple cognitive procedures, two which have been of particular interest to analysts:

1) grapheme-phoneme mapping where combinations of characters (graphemes) are mapped onto their related sound (phonemes) and which are thus "decoded".

2) visible word form acknowledgement for mapping of familiar words onto their mental representations. Collectively, these procedures allow us to pronounce words and access meaning. Relative to these cognitive procedures, studies in adults and children have exhibited that reading is backed with a network of areas in the still left hemisphere, like the occipito-temporal, temporo-parietal, and substandard frontal cortices. The occipito-temporal cortex keeps the "visible phrase form area". Both temporo-parietal and poor frontal cortices are likely involved in phonological and semantic digesting of

words, with poor frontal cortex also mixed up in formation of talk sound. These areas have been proven to change once we age group (Turkeltaub, et al., 2003) and are modified in people who have dyslexia (Richlan et al., 2011).

How about genes, brain chemistry, and brain function?

Several hereditary variants are associated with dyslexia, and their effect on the brain has been investigated in people and mice. Using pets which have been bred to have genes associated with dyslexia, experts are looking into how these genes might impact development-of and communication among brain location. These investigations dove-tail with studies in humans. Variations in brain anatomy (Darki, et al., 2012; Meda et al., 2008) and brain function (Deal et al., 2012; Pinel et al., 2012) have been seen in people who bring dyslexia-associated genes, even those who have good reading skills. Furthermore, to these investigations at the anatomical, physiological, and molecular levels, research workers want to pinpoint the chemical substance link with dyslexia. For instance, brain metabolites that are likely involved in allowing neurons to communicate can be visualized using another MRI-based technique called spectroscopy. Several metabolites (for example, choline) are usually different in people who have dyslexia (Pugh et al., 2014). Experts continue steadily to explore the connections between these results and are hopeful that what they learn will determine the sources of dyslexia. That is a difficult facet of research because distinctions in the brains of individuals with dyslexia aren't necessarily the reason for their reading issues (for example, it might also be considered a result of reading less).

What have brain images revealed about brain function in dyslexia?

Early functional studies were limited by adults because they employed invasive techniques that want radioactive materials. The field of brain mapping greatly benefited from the invention of fMRI. fMRI will not require the utilization of radioactive tracers for it to be safe for children and adults, and can be utilized frequently which facilitates longitudinal studies of development and involvement. First used to review dyslexia in 1996 (Eden et al., 1996), fMRI has since been trusted to review the brain's role in reading and its own components (phonology, orthography, and semantics). Studies from different countries have converged in results of modified left-hemisphere areas (Richlan et al., 2011), including ventral occipito-temporal, temporo-parietal, and second-rate frontal cortices (and their contacts). Results of the studies confirm the universality of dyslexia across different world dialects.

Changes in Reading, Changes in the Brain

Brain imaging research has revealed anatomical and functional changes in typically developing people as they figure out how to read (e.g. Turkeltaub et al., 2003); it is also revealed in children and adults with dyslexia pursuing effective reading education (Krafnick, et al., 2011; Eden et al., 2004). Such studies also shed light onto the brain-based variations of children with dyslexia who reap the benefits of reading instruction in comparison to those who neglect to make benefits. Neuroimaging data are also used to forecast long-term reading success for children with and without dyslexia.

What have brain images revealed about brain framework in dyslexia?

Evidence of a link between dyslexia and the framework of the brain was initially found out by examining the anatomy of brains of deceased adults who had dyslexia throughout their lifetimes. The left-greater-than-right asymmetry typically observed in the left hemisphere temporal lobe (planum temporale) had not been within these brains (Galaburda & Kemper, 1979), and ectopias (a displacement of brain cells to the top of brain) were mentioned (Galaburda, et al., 1985). Then researchers started to use MRI to find structural images in the brains of research volunteers with and without dyslexia. Current imaging techniques have exposed less grey and white matter quantity and changed white matter integrity in still left hemisphere occipito-temporal and temporo-parietal areas. Experts are still looking into how these results are influenced with a person's vocabulary and writing systems.

Causes vs Consequences

An important facet of research on the brain and reading is to determine if the findings will be the cause or the result of dyslexia. A number of the brain areas involved with dyslexia are also changed by understanding how to read, as shown by evaluations of adults who have been illiterate but learned to learn (Carreiras et al., 2009). Longitudinal studies in typical people uncover anatomical changes with age group, some of that are related to development (Giedd et al., 1999) as well as others to the firming up of vocabulary skills (Sowell et al., 2004) in correlation with improvements in phonological skills (Lu et al., 2007). Therefore, analysts are teasing aside the brain-based distinctions that may be noticed before children start to figure out how to read from variations that might occur due to less reading by people who have dyslexia. For instance, experts have found modified brain anatomy (Raschle, et al., 2011) and function (Raschle, et al., 2012) in pre-reading children with a family group background of dyslexia. Future studies using longitudinal designs (i.e., long-term), will inform the timeline of the changes and clarify cause and effects of anatomical and practical distinctions in dyslexia.

Chapter 5

Practical Brain Imaging Differences

One popular way for imaging brain function is **Functional Magnetic Resonance Imaging (fMRI)**, a non-invasive, relatively new method that steps physiological indicators of neural activation utilizing a strong magnet to pinpoint blood circulation. This method is named "practical" because individuals perform jobs while in (or under) the magnet, allowing dimension of the working brain as opposed to the activity of the brain at rest.

Several studies using useful imaging techniques that compared the brain activation patterns of readers with and without dyslexia show potentially important patterns of differences. We may expect that people with RD would show under-activation in areas where they may be weaker and over-activation in other areas, which is precisely what many experts have found (e.g., Shaywitz et al., 1998).

This sort of functional imaging research has just been utilized with children. That is partly because of the difficulties involved with imaging children, like the absolute dependence on the participant's check out to remain motionless through the scanning.

We will show the biggest, best-specified study for example of the new results with children. Shaywitz et al. (2002) researched one hundred and forty-four right handed children with and without RD on a number of in- and out-of-magnet duties; the likened brain activation between your two sets of children on jobs designed to faucet several component procedures of reading are:

- identifying the titles or seems of letters.

- sounding out non-sense words.

- sounding out and evaluating meanings of real words.

The non-impaired readers had more activation in every of the areas regarded to as very important to reading than the kids with dyslexia.

Shaywitz et al. (2002) also discovered that the children who have been good decoders experienced more activation in the areas very important to reading in the still left hemisphere and less in the right hemisphere than the kids with RD.

They suggested that for children with RD, disruption in the trunk reading systems in the left hemisphere that are crucial for skilled, fluent reading, leads the kids to compensate by using other, less efficient systems.

This finding could clarify the normal experience in school that even while children with dyslexia become accurate readers, their reading in grade-level text is often still slow and laboured with no fluency (e.g., Torgesen, Rashotte, & Alexander, 2001).

In summary, the brain of the person with dyslexia has a different distribution of metabolic activation than the brain of the person without reading problems when accomplishing the same vocabulary task. There's a failing of the left hemisphere back brain systems to operate properly during reading.

Furthermore, many people who have dyslexia often show greater activation in the low frontal regions of the brain. This leads to the final outcome that neural systems in frontal areas may compensate for the disruption in the posterior area (Shaywitz et al., 2003). These details often lead teachers to question whether brain imaging can be utilized as a diagnostic tool to recognize children with reading disabilities in college.

Can we display everyone that has reading difficulties?

Not yet. It really is an appealing eyesight of putting a kid we are worried about within an *fMRI machine* to quickly and accurately identify his/her problem, but research hasn't used it that much.

There are many explanations to why a clinical or school-based use of imaging ways to identify children with dyslexia is not presently feasible. *The first is the tremendous cost of fMRI machines, the computer systems, and the program needed to run them. Another area of the cost is the personnel that is required to run and interpret the results.*

Also, for this technology to be utilized for diagnosis, it requires to be accurate for people. Currently, email address details are reliable and reported for sets of participants; however, not necessarily for folks within each group (Richards, 2001; Shaywitz et al., 2002).

The amount of children who are identified to be average when they genuinely have a problem (false negatives), or as using a problem when these are average (false positives) would have to be significantly lower for imaging ways to be utilized for diagnosis of individual children.

Chapter 6

Strength of Dyslexic People

Seeing the larger picture

People who have dyslexia often see things more holistically. They skip the trees but start to see the forest.

"It's as though people who have dyslexia have a tendency to use a wide-angle zoom lens to take the world, while others have a tendency to use a telephoto; each is most beneficial at uncovering different types of fine details". *Matthew H. Schneps, Harvard University*

Finding the unusual one out

People who have dyslexia master global visual handling and the recognition of impossible statistics. Dyslexic scientist Christopher Tonkin explained his unusual level of sensitivity to "things out of place". Researchers in his type of work must seem sensible of enormous levels of visible data and accurately find dark hole anomalies.

There are more and more people with dyslexia in neuro-scientific astrophysics. It prompted research at the Harvard-Smithsonian Centre for Astrophysics. Results confirmed that people that have dyslexia are better at determining and memorizing complicated images.

Improved pattern recognition

People who have dyslexia are capable of observing how things hook up to form organic systems, and also to identify similarities among multiple things. Such advantages will tend to be of particular significance for areas like technology and mathematics, where visible representations are fundamental.

"I recognized I had dyslexia, and I quickly realized I had

formed this present for imaging. I reside in an environment of patterns and images, and I see things that nobody else sees. Due to dyslexia, I could see these patterns."

"You can't overcome it (dyslexia); you could work around it and make it happen for yourself, but it never goes away completely. That's probably a very important thing, because if dyslexia proceeded to go away, then your other presents would disappear completely too."

Good spatial knowledge

Many people who have dyslexia demonstrate better skills at manipulating 3D objects in their mind. Lots of the world's top architects and fashion designers have dyslexia.

Successful People with Dyslexia

"I had been called stupid. Not merely may I not read, but I couldn't memorize my assignment work. I used to be always in the bottom of the class. I became very depressed." **Richard Rogers**

"I performed poorly at college - once I attended, I was regarded to as stupid because of my dyslexia. I still have trouble reading. I must concentrate very hard at going still left to right, left to right; normally my vision just wanders underneath the web page." **Tommy Hilfiger**

Picture Thinkers

People who have dyslexia have a tendency to think in pictures rather than words. Research at the University or

College of California has proven children with dyslexia have improved picture recognition memory space.

Nineteenth-century French sculptor, Auguste Rodin, could stare at paintings in museums by day, and paint them from storage during the night. His dyslexia designed he could hardly read or write by age fourteen, along with his reading skills developing much later.

Sharper peripheral vision

People who have dyslexia have better peripheral eyesight than most, meaning they can easily take in a complete scene. Though it can be hard to target in on specific words, dyslexia appear to make it simpler to see external edges.

Business entrepreneurs

Did you know one in three American business owners

have dyslexia?

Business owners like **Thomas Edison, Henry Ford, Steve Jobs** and **Charles Schwab** were all dyslexic. Perhaps better strategic and creative considering could give a real business benefit.

"I appeared to think in different ways from my classmates. I had been very centred on trying to create a company and create something. My dyslexia led just how we communicated with customers." **Richard Branson**

Highly Creative

Lots of the world's most creative stars have dyslexia, such as **Johnny Depp, Keira Knighltly** and **Orlando Bloom**.

"Lots of the super developers I have met seemed to have a very important factor in keeping their experience from dyslexia." **Soren Petersen, Design Research Ph.D.**

Pablo Picasso (Designer)

Picasso was described by his educators as "having difficulty differentiating the orientation of characters". Picasso coloured his topics as he noticed them - sometimes out of order, backwards or ugly. His paintings confirmed the energy of his creativity, that was perhaps associated with the shortcoming to see written words properly.

Thinking beyond your package - problem solving

People that have dyslexia are popular for having unexpected leaps of insight that solve issues with an unorthodox approach.

That is an intuitive method of problem solving that can appear like daydreaming. Looking from the windows is how dyslexics work, allowing their brain slip into natural and simplicity around a problem to let contacts assemble.

Lightning Source UK Ltd.
Milton Keynes UK
UKHW020723130622
404345UK00010B/804